AF457618

Contents

What is a rainbow diet? 6

How to eat the rainbow 8

Track your rainbow diet 9

Red foods 9

Red vegetables 10

Red fruit 10

Orange foods 12

Orange vegetables 13

Orange fruits 13

Yellow foods 14

Yellow vegetables 14

Yellow fruit 15

Green foods 17

Green vegetables 17

Green fruit 18

Purple-blue foods 20

Purple vegetables 21

Purple fruit 21

Dark red 23

Fruits and veggies 24

White and brown 25

Fruits and veggies 26

Pros of eating the rainbow 28

Rainbow Diet Sample Menu Plan 29

Breakfast 30

Lunch or dinner 30

Snacks 31

RAINBOW DIET RECIPES 33

Rainbow cupcakes 33

Lucky Charms Treats 37

Rainbow Vanilla Cheesecake Bars 39

Rainbow Ice Cream Cake.................................. 43

Rainbow Candy Pops... 45

Rainbow Swirl Cupcakes.................................. 46

Tie Dye Cheesecake Bars................................. 50

Rainbow Muddy Buddies.................................. 54

Rainbow Fro-Yo Pops 57

Six Layer Rainbow Cake 59

RAINBOW BARS 64

RAINBOW VEGGIE FLATBREAD PIZZA 66

Simple Homemade Marshmallows.................. 68

EASY RAINBOW PASTA NOODLES.................. 71

TASTE THE RAINBOW JELLO 72

Rainbow Waffles.. 75

Rainbow Bundt Cake 77

Rainbow Spaghetti 80

Rainbow fudge 82

Rainbow Fruit Roll-Ups 86

Rainbow Crepe Cake 89

Rainbow Jell-O Poke Cake Recipe 93

Rainbow Chicken & Veggies 95

Rainbow sangria 98

Rainbow pizzas 100

Rainbow zebra cake 102

Rainbow fruit skewers 107

Layered rainbow salad pots 109

Stuffed rainbow baguette 112

Rainbow rippled meringues 114

What is a rainbow diet?

The rainbow diet is not a new idea, but it's newly popular. The idea behind it is that colourful vegetables and fruit contain specific micronutrients that support your health and combat biological stress with antioxidants and anti-inflammatory molecules.

This type of biological stress affects your body at a cellular level — you probably know it as "oxidative stress", which is caused by free radicals. Fortunately, the antioxidants in rainbow diet foods help the body to neutralise free radicals and stop them from damaging your cells.

Free radicals are generated by your metabolism (the sum of life-giving chemical reactions inside your cells) and your environment. Here are some common sources of free radicals in everyday life:

- Mitochondria
- Inflammation
- Exercise
- Cigarette smoke and air pollutants
- Pesticides, radiation, industrial solvents

The rainbow diet nutrients don't act directly on free radicals. Instead, they prompt your body's natural antioxidant mechanisms, which increases your natural ability to reduce oxidative stress. It also has a few other great benefits too.

Plant foods are full of fibre, and fibre is what keeps your digestive system running optimally. Plus, fibre and other plant nutrients are prebiotics: food molecules for your gut bacteria that also help keep you healthy.

How to eat the rainbow

The rainbow diet plan is a simple and easy way to clean up your diet without restricting yourself. The ultimate goal is to add 30+ different colourful fruit and vegetables to your meals every week.

That might sound like a lot, but it's not really. You just need to plan for one colourful plant food at every meal. Chances are, you'll probably end up adding more. Fresh and frozen fruit and vegetables are the best options, but in a pinch, canned is better than nothing.

Below, you'll find a rainbow diet chart for each colour. The rainbow food lists are divided by type: vegetable/fruit. We’ve also included links to our eat the rainbow guides by colour where you can get an in-depth profile of the nutrients by colour.

Track your rainbow diet

You can track your rainbow diet progress with the Atlas Health app on iOS and android. This food diary app uses image recognition tech to identify the ingredients of your meals from a photo, and it tracks your rainbow food goals!

Red foods

The red foods of the rainbow diet are rich in antioxidants and anti-inflammatory molecules that prevent inflammation and oxidative stress.

As you'll see below, you don't need a degree in food chemistry, because all these foods can all be found at the local supermarket.

Red vegetables

These red vegetables are really easy to get your hands on. You could try a rainbow diet breakfast of omelette with red pepper and red onion, or a rainbow diet lunch of open-faced rye sandwiches with smoked salmon and beetroot.

Red fruit

Red fruit are mouthwatering to look at and to taste thanks to the tart flavour of those healthful plant nutrients. Just add berries to your rainbow diet meal plan or top your morning porridge with pomegranate seeds for an extra boost.

Fruits and veggies

- tomatoes
- tomato paste
- tomato sauce
- watermelon
- pink guava
- grapefruit

Main phytonutrients

- lycopene (from the vitamin A family)

Main vitamins and minerals

- folate

- potassium
- vitamin A (lycopene)
- vitamin C
- vitamin K1

Health benefits

- anti-inflammatory
- antioxidant
- may benefit heart health
- may reduce sun-related skin damage
- may lower your risk of certain cancers

Orange foods

Orange food has similar phytonutrients to red rainbow foods, like beta-carotene, which give fruit and vegetables a rich orange-red hue. The benefits of orange fruits and vegetables also support reproductive health for men and women.

Orange vegetables

There's nothing groundbreaking about orange vegetables in the rainbow diet food chart. In fact, you've probably eaten some of them already this week. You can turbocharge your intake with delicious pumpkin soups, roasted sweet potatoes, and spices like turmeric.

Orange fruits

The rainbow diet food list of orange fruits is also inspiring and seasonal. Add cantaloupe and fresh apricots to your diet in summer, and citrus and persimmon in winter to boost your body's natural antioxidant mechanisms.

Yellow foods

Yellow foods are particularly good for your digestive tract. They contain prebiotics that encourage your gut bacteria to produce short-chain fatty acids — special molecules that nourish the cells of your gut.

Yellow vegetables

Put some sunshine in your belly with these cheerful yellow vegetables of the rainbow diet. Try some spiralised squash instead of pasta, or even a simple baked potato topped with some other lovely rainbow foods.

Yellow fruit

Yellow rainbow fruit like apples and Asian pears are excellent snack options. You can also diversify your palate with rainbow diet recipes for yellow foods, like a vegan pineapple "ice-cream" that uses a frozen banana as a base.

Fruits and veggies

- carrots
- sweet potatoes
- yellow peppers
- bananas
- pineapple

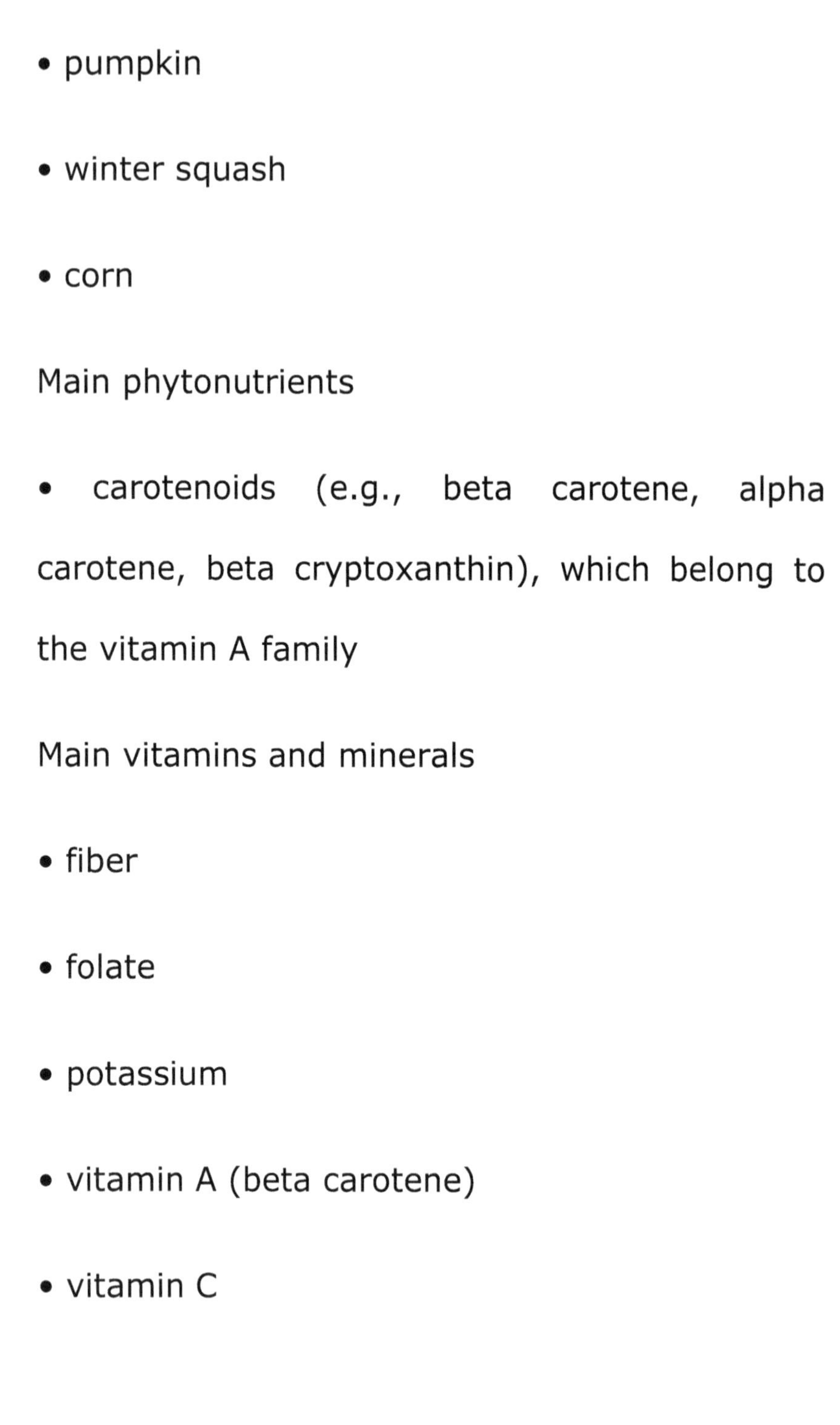

- tangerines
- pumpkin
- winter squash
- corn

Main phytonutrients

- carotenoids (e.g., beta carotene, alpha carotene, beta cryptoxanthin), which belong to the vitamin A family

Main vitamins and minerals

- fiber
- folate
- potassium
- vitamin A (beta carotene)
- vitamin C

Health benefits

- anti-inflammatory
- antioxidant
- may benefit heart health
- supports eye health
- may lower your risk of cancer

Green foods

Green foods of the rainbow diet contain nutrients that are particularly good at protecting your cardiovascular system from oxidative stress. In particular, oxidative stress has been linked to high blood pressure, atherosclerosis (the narrowing of your arteries), and heart disease.

Green vegetables

There are so many green rainbow vegetables that you are literally spoilt for choice. With a plethora of peas and leafy greens, not to mention avocado, broccoli, and artichokes, there's definitely something in there for everyone.

Green fruit

If you drink a cup of green tea and eat kiwis, then you're already on your way to achieving your rainbow food goals. Pears, limes, and olives also count as green rainbow foods that will titillate your taste buds.

Fruits and veggies

- spinach
- kale

- broccoli
- avocados
- asparagus
- green cabbage
- Brussels sprouts
- green herbs

Main phytonutrients

- Leafy greens: chlorophyll and carotenoids
- Cruciferous greens (e.g., broccoli, cabbage): indoles, isothiocyanates, glucosinolates

Main vitamins and minerals

- fiber
- folate

- magnesium
- potassium
- vitamin A (beta carotene)
- vitamin K1

Health benefits

- anti-inflammatory
- antioxidant
- cruciferous veggies, in particular, may lower your risk of cancer and heart disease

Purple-blue foods

Purple and blue rainbow foods share the same types of plant nutrients, which also give them their unique colour. Now, you might be wondering where on earth you'll find blue and purple vegetables and fruit, but when you see our list, you'll change your mind.

Purple vegetables

Start your dinner off with some beetroot-infused hummus and baba ghanoush for a prebiotic rainbow food twist on traditional Mediterranean dips. Roast some turnips, purple potatoes, and serve with purple cauliflower for your Sunday roast, and you're sorted!

Purple fruit

The rainbow food chart of purple fruit is short and sweet. You should have no trouble getting your hands on these beautiful berries, drupes, and grapes. They're delicious, which makes them a lovely and easy addition to your rainbow food diet!

Fruits and veggies

- blueberries
- blackberries
- Concord grapes
- red/purple cabbage
- eggplant
- plums
- elderberries

Main phytonutrients

- anthocyanins

Main vitamins and minerals

- fiber
- manganese

- potassium
- vitamin B6
- vitamin C
- vitamin K1

Health benefits

- anti-inflammatory
- antioxidant
- may benefit heart health
- may lower your risk of neurological disorders
- may improve brain function
- may lower your risk of type 2 diabetes
- may lower your risk of certain cancers

Dark red

Fruits and veggies

- beets
- prickly pears

Main phytonutrients

- betalains

Main vitamins and minerals

- fiber
- folate
- magnesium
- manganese
- potassium
- vitamin B6

Health benefits

- anti-inflammatory
- antioxidant
- may lower your risk of high blood pressure
- may benefit heart health
- may lower your risk of certain cancers
- may support athletic performance through increased oxygen uptake

White and brown

The foods belonging to this category might lack colour, but not nutrients. Be it providing calcium, proteins and healthy bacteria called probiotics in Greek Yogurt or Vitamin C, vitamin K, folate, and fiber in cauliflower, white foods like mushrooms, turnips, tofu, chickpeas and potatoes are packed with nutrients. They contain health promoting chemicals such as allicin and allinin, which help improve blood pressure, and lower total and LDL cholesterol levels.

Fruits and veggies

- cauliflower
- garlic
- leeks
- onions
- mushrooms
- daikon radish
- parsnips
- white potatoes

Main phytonutrients

- anthoxanthins (flavonols, flavones), allicin

Main vitamins and minerals

- fiber
- folate
- magnesium
- manganese
- potassium
- vitamin B6
- vitamin K1

Health benefits

- anti-inflammatory
- antioxidant
- may lower your risk of colon and other cancers
- may benefit heart health

Pros of eating the rainbow

Simply put, eating the rainbow involves eating fruits and vegetables of different colors every day.

Plants contain different pigments, or phytonutrients, which give them their color. Different-colored plants are linked to higher levels of specific nutrients and health benefits.

While eating more vegetables and fruit is always a good idea, focusing on eating a variety of colors will increase your intake of different nutrients to benefit various areas of your health.

While there are many purported benefits of phytonutrients, it's difficult to perform randomized controlled trials — the most rigorous type of research — to prove their efficacy. As such, most research is based on population-level intakes and disease risk.

That said, almost all studies show benefits from regularly eating colorful fruits and vegetables with virtually no downsides. By getting a variety of color in your diet, you're giving your body an array of vitamins, minerals, and phytochemicals to benefit your health

Rainbow Diet Sample Menu Plan

The great thing about eating the rainbow is it's easy to implement.

To eat the rainbow, try to incorporate two to three different-colored fruits or vegetables at every meal and at least one at every snack. While you don't have to eat every single color every day, try to get them into your diet a few times per week. Here are some ideas:

Breakfast

- an omelet with spinach, mushrooms, and orange bell peppers
- a smoothie with mango, banana, and dragonfruit
- a Greek yogurt bowl with blueberries, kiwi, and strawberries
- a breakfast egg sandwich with tomato, leafy greens, and avocado

Lunch or dinner

- a mixed salad with green cabbage, lettuce, apple, shredded carrots, red pepper, cucumbers, and cherry tomatoes paired with a protein source (e.g., kidney beans, chickpeas, grilled chicken, salmon)

- chicken with roasted sweet potatoes, Brussels sprouts, and garlic
- homemade soup with canned tomatoes, onion, garlic, chopped carrots, white potatoes or parsnip, and kale
- a goat cheese salad with pickled beets, arugula, avocado, and pecans
- spaghetti with tomato sauce, mushrooms, and zucchini

Snacks

- an apple with peanut butter
- red pepper slices with hummus
- grapes and cheese

- a green smoothie or juice
- a banana
- blueberries and yogurt
- broccoli, carrots, and dip
- dried mango slices
- 4–5 longan or lychee fruit
- edamame pods
- celery and melted cheese

The opportunities to include fruits and vegetables into your diet are endless. If you live in an area without fresh produce year-round, try purchasing frozen fruits and vegetables for some meals. They're equally nutritious, accessible, and affordable.

RAINBOW DIET RECIPES

The following recipes are rainbow-friendly while also being a treat to the taste buds. Try some of these rainbow diet recipes today.

Rainbow cupcakes

Prepartion time

50 minutes

Ingredients

- 110g unsalted butter , softened
- ½ tsp vanilla extract
- 110g caster sugar
- 2 large eggs

- 110g self-raising flour
- red, blue and yellow gel food colouring
- sprinkles (optional)

For the buttercream

- 150g butter , softened
- 300g icing sugar
- 3 tbsp milk

Instructions

1. Heat the oven to 180C/160C fan/gas 4 and fill a cupcake tray with 10 cases.

2. Beat the butter, vanilla and caster sugar together with an electric whisk until pale and fluffy.

3. Gradually whisk in the eggs, scraping down the sides of the bowl after each addition.

4. Mix in the flour and a pinch of salt until just combined.

5. Divide into five bowls and colour each a different shade with a drop of food colouring. We chose red, yellow, green, blue and purple.

6. Starting with the end of the rainbow (in our case purple), evenly spread 1 tsp of the mixture into each cupcake case using a piping bag or the back of a teaspoon. Top with 1 tsp of the next colour and spread – be careful not to mix the

colours together whilst bringing the mix all the way to the edge of the case.

7. Repeat until all the colours are used up and you're left with an even layer of red on the top.

8. Bake for 15 mins, until a skewer inserted into the middle of each cake comes out clean.

9. Leave to cool completely on a wire rack.

10. To make the buttercream, beat the butter until very soft.

11. Add the icing sugar, vanilla extract and a pinch of salt and whisk together until smooth (start off slowly to avoid an icing sugar cloud).

12. Beat in the milk until combined.

13. Pipe the buttercream on top of the cupcakes using a circular nozzle, or spread on with a palette knife.

14. Top with sprinkles, if you like.

Lucky Charms Treats

Prepartion time

1 hour

INGREDIENTS

- 1/2 c. (1 stick) butter, plus more for pan
- 1 (12-oz.) bag mini marshmallows
- 1/2 tsp. kosher salt
- 6 c. Lucky Charms

Instructions

1. Grease a 9"-x-9" baking dish with butter. In a large pot over medium heat, melt butter.
2. Add marshmallows and salt and stir until completely melted.
3. Remove from heat and stir in Lucky Charms.
4. Pour into pan and smooth top, being careful not to pack cereal too tightly into prepared dish.
5. Let cool completely before slicing and serving.

Rainbow Vanilla Cheesecake Bars

Prepartion time

4 hours

INGREDIENTS

FOR CRUST:

- Cooking spray, for pan
- 9 graham crackers, crushed
- 6 tbsp. butter, melted
- 1/4 c. sugar

FOR FILLING:

- 2 8-oz. blocks cream cheese, softened
- 1/4 c. sour cream
- 2/3 c. sugar
- 3 large eggs
- 1 tsp. pure vanilla extract
- 1 tsp. kosher salt
- Neon food dye in 6 colors

Instructions

1. Preheat oven to 325° and grease an 8"-x-8" pan with cooking spray.

2. Make crust: Add crushed graham crackers to a bowl with butter and sugar and mix until combined.

3. Press tightly into prepared pan.

4. Make filling: In a large bowl, beat together cream cheese, sour cream, and sugar until smooth.

5. Add eggs, vanilla, and salt and beat until combined. Pour about half the cheesecake mixture into pan and set aside.

6. Divide remaining mixture between six small bowls (or one bowl for each color you're using) and add a couple drops of food coloring to each bowl.

7. Stir to combine, adjusting color as desired.

8. Add spoonfuls of the dyed cheesecake mixture to the plain cheesecake mixture, alternating colors until you’ve used up the whole mixture.

9. Swirl colors together with a butter knife.

10. Place baking pan in a large roasting pan and pour in enough boiling water to come halfway up your baking pan.

11. Bake until only slightly jiggly, about 45 minutes.

12. Turn off oven and prop oven door open slightly.

13. Let cool in oven 1 hour. Remove pan from water and refrigerate until firm, 3 hours, or up to overnight.

14. Slice into bars and serve.

Rainbow Ice Cream Cake

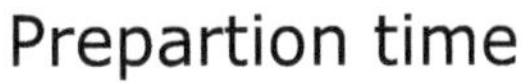

Prepartion time

5 hours 20 minutes

INGREDIENTS

- 3 c. heavy cream
- 1 14-oz. can sweetened condensed milk
- 1 tsp. pure vanilla extract
- Red, orange, yellow, green, blue, and purple food coloring

Instructions

1. In a large bowl using a hand mixer, beat heavy cream until medium peaks form.

2. Fold in sweetened condensed milk and vanilla until totally combined, then divide mixture among six bowls.

3. Add a different color food coloring to each bowl and mix thoroughly.

4. Spray a loaf pan with nonstick cooking spray and line with a large piece of plastic wrap.

5. Layer colors in order from red to purple, making sure to spread to the outer edges of the loaf pan.

6. When all colors have been used, freeze until firm, about 5 hours.

7. When ready to serve, take out of the freezer and remove from loaf pan. Slice and serve.

Rainbow Candy Pops

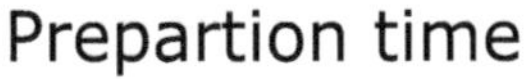

Prepartion time

10 minutes

INGREDIENTS

- 6 rainbow rope candies
- 2 c. sprite
- 1/4 c. vodka

Instructions

1. Cut each rope into 4 to 5 small pieces.
2. Twist each section three or four times then press together the ends until they stick.

3. Place in popsicle mold and repeat about 4 times, until the entire popsicle mold is filled with candy.

4. Fill each mold with Sprite and vodka.

5. Freeze until solid.

Rainbow Swirl Cupcakes

Prepartion time

1 hour

INGREDIENTS

FOR THE CUPCAKES

- 1 box vanilla cake mix, plus ingredients called for on box
- food coloring (red, yellow, green, blue)

FOR THE FROSTING

- 1 c. butter, softened
- 4 c. powdered sugar
- 1 tsp. pure vanilla extract
- 3 tbsp. heavy cream
- 1/8 tsp. kosher salt

Instructions

Make the cupcakes:

1. Prepare cake batter according to box instructions.

2. Divide batter into five bowls.

3. Add a few drops of red into one bowl, yellow in the second, green in the third, blue in the fourth, and two drops blue plus two drops red into the fifth.

4. Stir each bowl, adjusting the amount of food coloring you want until you have five colors of cake batter.

5. Spray a muffin tin with cooking spray or line with cupcake liners.

6. Spoon a little of each color batter into each cup of the tin, until they're filled two-thirds of the way up.

7. Bake according to box instructions. Set aside to cool.

8. Make the frosting: In a large bowl using a hand mixer or in the bowl of a stand mixer using the whisk attachment, beat butter until fluffy.

9. Add sugar, beating on low until combined, then whip in vanilla, heavy cream and salt. (Add more heavy cream, 1 tablespoon at a time, if you'd like a thinner consistency.)

10. Divide frosting into five bowls, adding food coloring to each and stirring, like you did with the cake batter.

11. Place each color in a resealable sandwich bag and snip off one corner.

12. Lay out a piece of plastic wrap.

13. Use each bag to pipe out a line of frosting in each color, side by side.

14. Roll up the plastic wrap, creating a tube of frosting. Twist the ends closed, then slip a star tip on one end.

15. Trim the plastic wrap that sticks through the star tip. Pipe onto cooled cupcakes.

Tie Dye Cheesecake Bars

Prepartion time

4 hours

INGREDIENTS

FOR THE CRUST

- 9 graham crackers
- 6 tbsp. butter, melted
- 1/4 c. sugar

FOR THE CHEESECAKE

- 2 8-oz. blocks cream cheese, softened
- 1/4 c. sour cream
- 3/4 c. sugar
- 2 large eggs
- 1/2 tsp. pure vanilla extract

- kosher salt
- Neon food dye in four colors

Instructions

1. Preheat oven to 325° and line a 8"-x-8" pan with parchment paper.

2. Make crust: In a food processor fitted with a metal blade, blend graham crackers until fine crumbs form, then add to a bowl with butter and sugar and mix until combined.

3. Press tightly into prepared pan.

4. Make filling: In a large bowl, beat together cream cheese, sour cream, and sugar until smooth. Add eggs, vanilla, and salt and beat until combined.

5. Divide mixture between four small bowls (or one bowl for each color you're using) and add a couple drops of food coloring to each bowl.

6. Stir to combine, adjusting color as desired.

7. Add spoonfuls of the dyed cheesecake mixture to graham cracker crust, alternating colors until you’ve used up the whole mixture.

8. Swirl colors together with a knife.

9. Bake until only slightly jiggly, about 40 minutes.

10. Let cool slightly, then refrigerate until firm, 3 hours, or up to overnight.

11. Slice into bars and serve.

Rainbow Muddy Buddies

Prepartion time

25 minutes

INGREDIENTS

- 6 c. Chex cereal
- 1 c. semisweet chocolate chips
- 1/2 c. creamy peanut butter
- 1/2 c. butter, divided
- 1 1/2 c. powdered sugar
- 2 c. white chocolate chips
- food coloring (pink, purple, blue, green)
- 1/2 c. Lucky Charms

- rainbow sprinkles

Instructions

1. In a microwave-safe bowl, combine chocolate chips, peanut butter and 1/4 c butter.

2. Microwave for 30 seconds, stir, then microwave again for 30 seconds, stirring until chips are fully melted and combined.

3. Pour mixture over cereal, stirring to combine, then place in a gallon-sized resealable bag.

4. Add powdered sugar, seal bag and toss to coat.

5. Spread mixture on a wax paper-covered baking sheet. Set aside.

6. In a large microwave-safe bowl, combine remaining butter and white chocolate chips.

7. Microwave in 30-second intervals, stirring in between, until chips are fully melted.

8. Divide white chocolate into five bowls.

9. Add 2-3 drops of food coloring to each bowl, creating pink, green, yellow and blue white chocolate.

10. For the fifth bowl, combine 2 drops pink and 2 drops blue food coloring, stirring until it's purple.

11. Drizzle various colors of white chocolate on top of the Muddy Buddies, creating a rainbow effect.

12. Top with Lucky Charms and sprinkles.

13. Let cool in refrigerator for at least 10 minutes.

14. Break apart and serve.

Rainbow Fro-Yo Pops

Prepartion time

4 hours 30 minutes

INGREDIENTS

- 1 c. frozen raspberries
- 1 c. frozen strawberries
- 1 c. Frozen Mango
- 1 c. frozen blueberries
- 1 1/2 c. frozen pineapple
- 1 c. baby spinach
- 3 c. Vanilla Greek yogurt

Instructions

1. In a blender or food processor, blend 1 cup fruit with 1/2 cup yogurt until combined (cleaning out processor between colors).

2. For the spinach, blend with remaining 1/2 cup frozen pineapple.

3. Transfer to bowls.

4. Layer 1/4" of each color in popsicle molds in the shades of a rainbow.

5. Insert popsicle sticks and freeze until firm, 4 hours.

6. Run popsicle molds under warm water for 20 seconds for easy removal.

Six Layer Rainbow Cake

Prepartion time

40 minutes

Ingredients

for the cake:

- 4 1/2 cups flour
- 1 1/2 tablespoons baking powder
- 1 teaspoon salt
- 1 1/2 cups butter, room temperature
- 3 cups sugar
- 6 large eggs, room temperature
- 1 teaspoon vanilla
- 1 1/2 cups buttermilk
- food coloring

for the frosting:

- 4 sticks unsalted butter

- 4 cups confectioners' sugar
- pinch of salt
- 3 tablespoons heavy cream
- 2 teaspoons vanilla
- food coloring (if desired)

Instructions

1. Preheat oven to 350. Butter and flour 8-inch cake pans (as many as you have!) and set aside. In a medium bowl, whisk together flour, baking powder, and salt, and set aside.

2. In a large bowl or the bowl of a stand mixer, beat butter and sugar until light and fluffy.

3. Add the eggs one at a time, mixing well after each addition, then add the vanilla.

4. Add the flour mixture in three additions, alternating with the buttermilk, and beginning and ending with the flour.

5. Divide the cake batter into sixths in six different bowls, and add a different color of food coloring to each bowl. I used gel food coloring and used about a dime sized amount for each bowl.

6. Bake in preheated oven 20-25 minutes, or until a toothpick inserted in the center comes out clean.

7. Repeat with remaining batter, and let all layers cool completely.

8. To make the frosting, beat the butter until light and fluffy.

9. Add the confectioners' sugar and salt, and beat to combine.

10. Add the heavy cream and vanilla and beat until light and fluffy.

11. Add food coloring if desired (I added a very small amount of blue food coloring).

12. To assemble, level each layer of cake.

13. Stack the layers, adding a small amount of buttercream between each layer to hold them together.

14. Frost with remaining buttercream and enjoy!

RAINBOW BARS

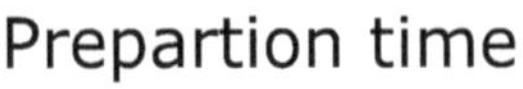

Prepartion time

20 minutes

Ingredients

- 6 tablespoons margarine (works much better than butter for this recipe)
- 16 ounces mini marshmallows
- 12 cups Fruit Loops

Instructions

1. Line a 9 x 13 pan with parchment paper and spray with a non-stick spray.

2. Melt margarine in a large pot over medium heat.

3. Add marshmallow and stir until melted and smooth.

4. Remove from heat. (Don't over heat the marshmallows. It can cause the cereal to become soggy)

5. Add Fruit Loops and stir until evenly coated with marshmallow.

6. Press into pan using greased parchment paper.

7. Chill until set. Cut into yummy bars.

RAINBOW VEGGIE FLATBREAD PIZZA

Prepartion time

30 minutes

Ingredients

- 1 package (2-piece) Stonefire naan
- 1/2 cup pizza sauce, homemade or store-bought
- 1/2 cup shredded part-skim Mozzarella cheese
- about 4 cups chopped colorful veggies (I used broccoli florets, green peppers, yellow peppers, orange peppers, grape tomatoes, red onions and thinly-sliced purple potatoes)
- 2 tsp. olive oil

- 1 tsp. Italian seasonings
- (optional toppings: grated Parmesan cheese, red pepper flakes)

INSTRUCTIONS

1. Preheat oven to 425 degrees F.
2. Lay out both pieces of naan in a single layer on a large baking sheet.
3. Divide pizza sauce between the two pieces of naan, and use a spoon to spread it over the top of the naan.
4. Sprinkle the cheese on top of the pizza sauce.
5. Then layer the veggies in a rainbow pattern on top of the cheese.

6. Drizzle or mist each pizza with a bit of olive oil.

7. Then sprinkle each pizza with the Italian seasonings.

8. Bake for about 20 minutes, or until the veggies are cooked and the crust is slightly golden.

9. Remove pizzas from oven, and sprinkle with optional toppings if desired.

10. Slice and serve warm.

Simple Homemade Marshmallows

Prepartion time

25 minutes

Ingredients

- 1 1/2 cups water
- 3 envelopes unflavored gelatin (about 2 teaspoons per packet)
- 2 1/4 cups sugar, granulated
- 1 teaspoon vanilla extract
- Powdered Sugar for tossing, optional

Instructions

1. In a medium saucepan on the stove, add water and sprinkle gelatin over
2. Let set 1 minute
3. Add sugar and vanilla, stir to combine

4. Heat mixture just until sugar is dissolved, about 3-4 minutes

5. Remove from heat and let cool until you can almost hold your hand on the side of pan

6. Transfer to stand mixer and beat on high speed for 15-20 minutes until stiff peaks form

7. Transfer to 13x9 pan and chill at least 2 hours or overnight

8. For colored marshmallows - divide batter and add coloring

9. Pour into pan and spread evenly

10. Cut into 1 inch squares. Toss in Powdered Sugar if desired.

EASY RAINBOW PASTA NOODLES

Prepartion time

20 minutes

INGREDIENTS

- Spaghetti Noodles (or any type of pasta)
- Liquid Food Coloring
- Ziploc Bags
- Water

Instructions

1. Cook the spaghetti noodles al dente, according to package directions and strain.

2. You'll need one Ziploc bag for each color of pasta you want to make.

3. Add two tablespoons of warm water to each bag and add about 20 drops of food coloring to the water.

TASTE THE RAINBOW JELLO

Prepartion time

2 hours 30 minutes

INGREDIENTS

- 3 ounces red jello cherry or strawberry
- 3 ounces orange jello
- 3 ounces yellow jello lemon
- 3 ounces green jello lime
- 3 ounces blue jello
- 3 ounces purple jello grape
- 16 ounces cool whip

INSTRUCTIONS

1. Prepare purple (or whatever color you want on the bottom) jello as directed, using the "quick chill" method, meaning add some ice.

2. Pour jello into glasses, (or a 9'x13' baking dish sprayed lightly with cooking spray), reserving about 1/3 of the liquid jello.

3. Put glasses, or dish in the refrigerator and chill for 15-30 minutes, or until slightly set.

4. Mix about 1/3 cup of cool whip into the remaining purple jello.

5. Pour the jello/cool whip mixture on top of the slightly set purple jello already in the glasses (or dish).

6. Repeat process for each color.

7. Once set, top with some additional cool whip and sprinkles if desired.

Rainbow Waffles

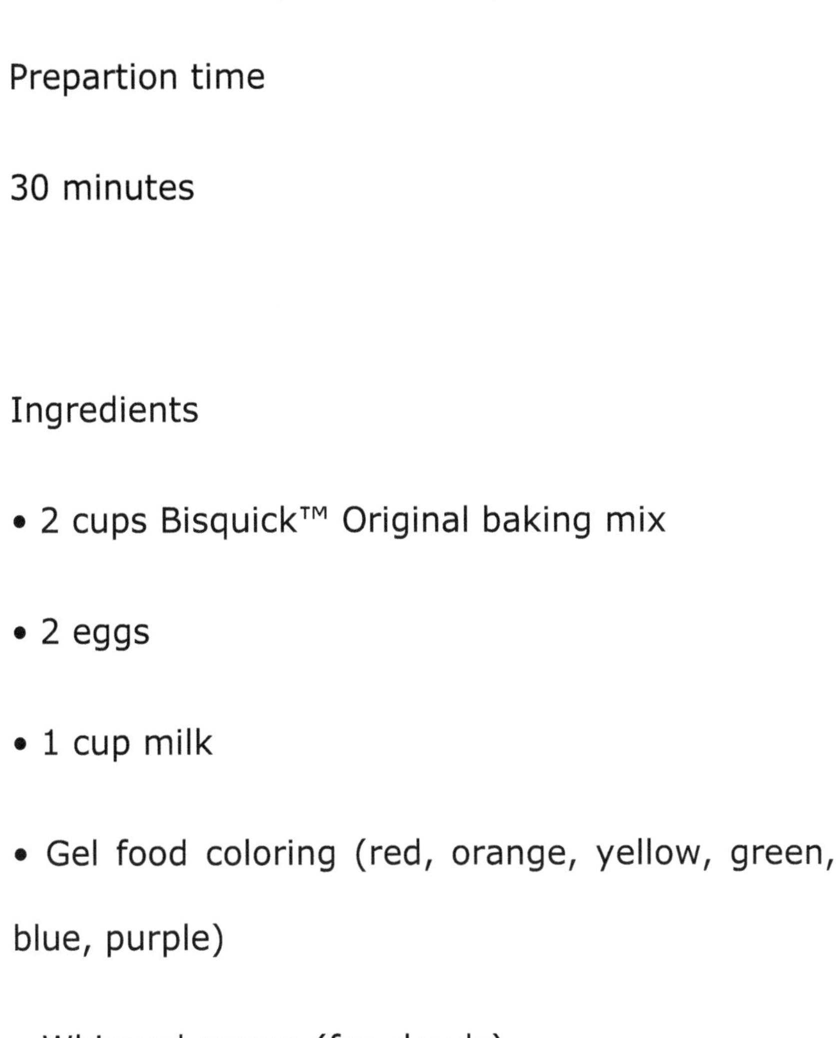

Prepartion time

30 minutes

Ingredients

- 2 cups Bisquick™ Original baking mix
- 2 eggs
- 1 cup milk
- Gel food coloring (red, orange, yellow, green, blue, purple)
- Whipped cream (for clouds)
- Lucky Charms™ cereal (for the treasure)

Instructions

1. In a large bowl, whisk together Bisquick™, eggs and milk until smooth.

2. Divide the batter into six portions, around 1/3 cup each, giving a little extra to the bowls for the red and orange colors.

3. Use gel food coloring (red, orange, yellow, green, blue, purple) to color each bowl of batter to your desired vibrancy.

4. Whisk in food coloring until evenly blended.

5. Transfer each color of batter to its own piping bag and cut off the tips (careful not to spill the batter).

6. Carefully pour each color into a heated circle waffle maker to make your rainbow, starting

with red, then orange, yellow, green, blue and purple.

7. Cook according to waffle maker instructions.

8. Remove, and repeat with remaining batter.

9. Cut each waffle in half.

10. Serve with whipped cream for clouds and Lucky Charms™ as the treasure at the end of the rainbow.

Rainbow Bundt Cake

Prepartion time

5 minutes

INGREDIENTS

- 1 box vanilla cake mix, plus ingredients called for on box
- Red food coloring
- Yellow food coloring
- Green food coloring
- Blue food coloring
- Purple food coloring
- 1 1/2 c. powdered sugar
- 2 tbsp. heavy cream
- Gold sanding sugar, for decorating

Instructions

1. Preheat oven to 350°.

2. Grease a bundt pan with cooking spray.

3. In a large bowl, prepare cake batter according to package directions.

4. Divide batter between 5 bowls.

5. Using food coloring, dye each bowl of batter a different color, being sure to stir well.

6. Pour red batter into bottom of greased bundt pan, then carefully pour yellow batter on top, trying to create an even layer and not mix together the batters.

7. Repeat with green, blue and then purple.

8. Bake until a toothpick inserted in the middle comes out clean, about 35 minutes.

9. Cool for 10 minutes in pan, then carefully invert cake onto a cooling rack to cool completely.

10. In a small bowl, whisk together powdered sugar and heavy cream until smooth.

11. Drizzle over cooled cake, then sprinkle with gold sanding sugar.

Rainbow Spaghetti

Prepartion time

20 minutes

INGREDIENTS

- 6 Ziploc bags
- 1 lb. spaghetti, cooked
- Food coloring (we used 6)
- 1 c. Water, Divided
- 3 tbsp. butter, melted
- 1/3 c. freshly grated Parmesan
- kosher salt
- Freshly ground black pepper

Instructions

1. Place 2 tbsp water into each ziplock back (we used 6 for 6 different colors).

2. Add 10 drops gel food coloring to each bag.

3. Divide the spaghetti into the 6 different bags.

4. Shake until they are coated in their colors.

5. Remove each pasta individually from ziplock bag and rinse with cold water.

6. Combine in a large bowl and toss together with butter and parm.

7. Season with salt and pepper and serve.

Rainbow fudge

Prepartion time

5 hours 10 minutes

INGREDIENTS

- 3 c. white chocolate chips
- 1 14-oz. can sweetened condensed milk
- 1 tbsp. butter
- 1/2 tsp. almond extract
- Red, orange, yellow, green, blue, and purple food coloring

Instructions

1. Lightly grease an 8"-x-8″ pan with cooking spray and line with parchment paper.

2. In a medium saucepan over medium-low heat, combine white chocolate, sweetened condensed milk, and butter.

3. Stir often, until melted and smooth, then stir in almond extract.

4. Divide mixture between 6 bowls.

5. Add a different color food coloring to each bowl, and stir until combined.

6. Cover each bowl with plastic until ready to use.

7. Spread the purple mixture into the prepared loaf pan and freeze until solid, about 10 minutes.

8. In a separate 8"-x-8” pan lined with parchment paper, spread the blue mixture into

in even layer and freeze until solid, about 10 minutes.

9. Invert the blue layer onto the purple.

10. Repeat with remaining colors, following the order of the rainbow, freezing between each layer.

11. Refrigerate until solid, about 4 hours. Invert onto a cutting board, peel off parchment paper and slice fudge into small squares.

12. Store in an airtight container in the refrigerator until ready to eat.

Rainbow Fruit Roll-Ups

Prepartion time

3 hours 15 minutes

INGREDIENTS

- 8 oz. strawberries, rinsed, dried, trimmed, and halved
- 5 tsp. freshly squeezed lemon juice, divided
- 4 1/2 tsp. sugar, divided
- 6 oz. blueberries, rinsed and dried
- 6 oz. raspberries, rinsed and dried
- 6 oz. blackberries, rinsed and dried
- 2 medium, ripe champagne mangoes, peeled and chopped

Instructions

1. Preheat oven to 170°.

2. Line three large rimmed baking sheets with parchment paper and lightly grease with cooking spray.

3. In a food processor or blender, purée strawberries with 1 teaspoon lemon juice and 1 teaspoon sugar until smooth.

4. Transfer to a bowl.

5. Repeat process with blueberries, raspberries, and blackberries. (If desired, strain raspberries and blackberries and discard seeds.)

6. Repeat again with mango, adding final teaspoon lemon juice and 1/2 teaspoon sugar.

7. Carefully pour purées onto baking sheets next to each other, in horizontal lines, spreading thin (until almost transparent) with a spoon so all colors are an even thickness.

8. Bake until dried out and no longer sticky, 3 to 4 hours.

9. Using scissors or a sharp paring knife, cut leather into vertical strips and roll up.

Rainbow Crepe Cake

Prepartion time

1 hour 10 minutes

INGREDIENTS

FOR THE CREPES

- 1 c. whole milk
- 1/2 c. heavy cream
- 1 c. all-purpose flour
- 1/4 c. powdered sugar
- 1/4 tsp. kosher salt
- 4 large eggs
- 3 tbsp. butter, melted

- rainbow food coloring

FOR WHIPPED CREAM

1. 2 c. heavy cream, chilled
2. 1/4 c. powdered sugar
3. 1/2 tsp. pure vanilla extract

Instructions

1. In a blender, combine milk, heavy cream, flour, powdered sugar, salt, eggs and butter.
2. Blend until mixture is smooth and foamy. If possible, let batter sit for 15 minutes at room temperature (or up to overnight in the fridge).

3. Divide the crepe batter between 6 bowls (one for every color), and dye each bowl of batter a different color of the rainbow.

4. Heat a medium nonstick skillet over medium heat.

5. Lightly coat with more butter or vegetable oil.

6. Add about one-quarter to one-third cup batter and swirl the batter to completely cover bottom of skillet.

7. Cook until the bottom of the crepe is set, 2 to 3 minutes.

8. Using a rubber spatula (or chopsticks) loosen edge of crepe then quickly flip.

9. Cook for 1 minute more then slide crepe out of skillet on a cooling rack to cool.

10. Repeat with remaining batters, adding more butter or oil to the pan as necessary.

11. Each color batter should yield about 5 crepes.

12. Make whipped cream: In a large bowl using a hand mixer or in the bowl of a stand mixer using the whisk attachment, combine heavy cream, powdered sugar and vanilla and beat until soft peaks form.

13. Assemble crepe cake: Lay 1 purple crepe on a cake plate.

14. Using an offset spatula, cover with a thin layer of whipped cream, leaving a 1/4" border.

15. Cover with another purple crepe and repeat to make a purple stack.

16. Repeat process with other rainbow colors.

Rainbow Jell-O Poke Cake Recipe

Prepartion time

2 hours

INGREDIENTS

- 1 box vanilla cake mix
- 1 package cherry Jell-O
- 1 package blue raspberry Jell-O
- 2 c. boiling water
- 2 c. cold water
- 1 container whipped topping

- rainbow sprinkles

Instructions

1. Prepare the vanilla cake according to the package's instructions, then let it cool for at least 20 minutes before poking the top of the entire cake with the handle of a wooden spoon.

2. Pour the cherry Jell-O mix into one bowl, and the blue raspberry Jell-O mix into another bowl.

3. Add a cup of boiling water to each bowl and whisk until the Jell-O powder has dissolved.

4. Stir a cup of cold water into each bowl.

5. Immediately pour both flavors of Jell-O onto the cake, filling alternate holes and areas of the cake to create a spotted or tie-dye effect.

6. Refrigerate for two hours.

7. Top the cake with a layer of whipped topping and cover with sprinkles.

Rainbow Chicken & Veggies

Prepartion time

45 minutes

INGREDIENTS

- 2 c. cherry tomatoes
- 3 c. baby carrots
- 2 yellow bell peppers, thinly sliced
- 1 large head broccoli, florets removed

- 2 small red onions, cut into wedges
- 1 lb. boneless skinless chicken breasts, cubed
- 2 c. cooked brown rice

FOR THE MARINADE

- 1/3 c. extra-virgin olive oil
- Juice of 2 limes
- 1/4 c. freshly chopped cilantro
- kosher salt
- Freshly ground black pepper

Instructions

1. Preheat oven to 400º.

2. On two large sheet pans, place tomatoes, carrots, bell peppers, broccoli, red onion, and chicken.

3. Make marinade: In a medium bowl, combine olive oil, lime juice, and cilantro and season with salt and pepper.

4. Whisk until combined.

5. Pour marinade over veggies and chicken and season with more salt and pepper.

6. Toss until completely combined.

7. Bake until vegetables are tender and chicken is cooked through, 25 minutes.

8. Divide cooked rice among five containers and top with roasted veggies and chicken. (Note:

Cooked poultry stays good in the fridge for 3 to 4 days.

9. We recommend freezing your Thursday and Friday meals for best results.)

Rainbow sangria

Prepartion time

20 minutes

INGREDIENTS

- 1 1/2 bottles moscato, chilled
- 1/2 c. triple sec
- Juice of 3 limes

- 1/4 c. granulated sugar
- 3 c. blackberries
- 3 c. blueberries
- 6 kiwis, peeled and sliced
- 2 c. diced pineapple
- 2 c. diced mango
- 2 c. halved strawberries

Instructions

1. In a large pitcher, stir together white wine, triple sec, lime juice, and sugar until combined.
2. In tall glasses, layer blackberries, blueberries, kiwis, pineapple, mango, and strawberries.
3. Pour wine mixture over fruit and serve.

Rainbow pizzas

Prepartion time

40 minutes

Ingredients

- 2 plain pizza bases
- 6 tbsp passata
- 400g mixed red and yellow tomatoes , sliced
- 75g sprouting broccoli , stems finely sliced
- 8 green olives , pitted and halved (optional)
- 150g mozzarella cherries (bocconcini)

- 2 tbsp fresh pesto
- handful fresh basil leaves, to serve

Instructions

1. Heat the oven to 180C/160C fan/gas 4.
2. Put each pizza base on a baking sheet and spread each with half of the passata.
3. Arrange the tomatoes on the top in rings or wedges of colour and add the broccoli and the olives, if using.
4. Squish the mozzarella cherries (bocconcini) a little before dotting them over the pizzas, then drizzle 1 tbsp pesto over each.
5. Bake for 15-20 mins or until the top is bubbling and just starting to brown a little.

6. Scatter over the basil leaves before serving.

Rainbow zebra cake

Prepartion time

1 hour 20 minutes

Ingredients

- 375g salted butter , softened, plus extra for the tin
- 375g golden caster sugar
- 6 large eggs , at room temperature
- 375g self-raising flour
- 1½ tsp baking powder

- 150ml milk
- blue and pink food colouring (see tip, below)
- sprinkles , to decorate

For the icing

- 250g salted butter , softened
- 400g icing sugar , sifted
- vanilla pod, seeds scraped out
- 100g full-fat cream cheese

Instructions

1. Heat the oven to 180C/160C fan/gas 4.

2. Butter and line three 20cm loose-bottomed sandwich cake tins with baking parchment.

3. To make the sponge, beat the butter and sugar together in a stand mixer or using an electric whisk for 5-8 mins or until light and fluffy.

4. Whisk in the eggs, one at a time, beating well after each addition.

5. Fold in the flour, baking powder and milk to loosen.

6. Divide the mixture between three mixing bowls, weighing for accuracy if you like.

7. Colour one of the batters blue and another pink, starting with a little colouring, then adding more for a deeper finish.

8. Leave one of the bowls of batter uncoloured.

9. Get the three cake tins and bowls of batter ready in front of you.

10. Spoon a heaped tablespoon of blue batter into the centre of the first tin, then pink in the second, and plain in the third.

11. Working quickly so that it doesn't spread too much, add another dollop of a different coloured batter on top of each one.

12. Don't wait for the batter to settle or spread, just keep alternating the colours until you run out.

13. The weight of each layer will cause the batter to spread as you go, so very gently tap and shake the cake tins to even out the mixture,

then bake in the centre of the oven for 25-30 mins or until firm to the touch.

14. Turn out top-side down onto wire racks straightaway, then leave to cool completely.

15. For the icing, put the butter, icing sugar and vanilla seeds into a stand mixer fitted with the paddle attachment or put in a bowl and use an electric whisk.

16. Beat for 5 mins or until fluffy and aerated.

17. Add the cream cheese and beat briefly until just combined.

18. Place one of the cakes on a cake stand or serving plate and spread 2 tbsp of the buttercream on top, then repeat with the other sponges.

19. Spread a smooth layer of the icing over the top and sides of the cake, using a large palette knife, leaving some slightly less iced spots for a 'naked' finish.

20. Top with sprinkles and candles, if you like. Will keep in an airtight tin for three days.

Rainbow fruit skewers

Prepartion time

15 minutes

Ingredients

- 7 raspberries
- 7 hulled strawberries

- 7 tangerine segments
- 7 cubes peeled mango
- 7 peeled pineapple chunks
- 7 peeled kiwi fruit chunks
- 7 green grapes
- 7 red grapes
- 14 blueberries

Instructions

1. Take 7 wooden skewers and thread the following fruit onto each – 1 raspberry, 1 hulled strawberry, 1 tangerine segment, 1 cube of peeled mango, 1 chunk of peeled pineapple, 1

chunk of peeled kiwi, 1 green and 1 red grape, and finish off with 2 blueberries.

2. Arrange in a rainbow shape and let everyone help themselves.

Layered rainbow salad pots

Prepartion time

37 minutes

Ingredients

- 350g pasta shapes (De Cecco is a good brand that stays nice and firm)

- 200g green beans , trimmed and chopped into short lengths
- 160g can tuna in olive oil, drained
- 4 tbsp mayonnaise
- 4 tbsp natural yogurt
- ½ small pack chives , snipped (optional)
- 200g cherry tomatoes , quartered
- 1 orange pepper , cut into little cubes 195g can sweetcorn, drained

Instructions

1. Cook the pasta until it is still a little al dente (2 mins less than the pack instructions) and drain well.

2. Cook the green beans in simmering water for 2 mins, then rinse in cold water and drain well.

3. Mix the tuna with the mayonnaise and yogurt.

4. Add the chives, if using.

5. Tip the pasta into a large glass bowl or four small ones, or four wide-necked jars (useful for taking on picnics).

6. Spoon the tuna dressing over the top of the pasta.

7. Add a layer of green beans, followed by a layer of cherry tomatoes, then the pepper and sweetcorn.

8. Cover and chill until you're ready to eat.

Stuffed rainbow baguette

Prepartion time

10 minutes

Ingredients

- 1 artisan-style baguette
- 4 tbsp hummus
- 8 slices medium cheddar
- ¼ red pepper , thinly sliced
- ¼ cooked beetroot , shredded
- 2 radishes , thinly sliced
- 1 yellow or orange carrot , shredded or grated

- handful green leaves
- 1 tbsp vegetarian pesto , mixed with 1 tbsp olive oil

Instructions

1. Cut the baguette in half so you can open it out like a book.
2. Spread the hummus over the bottom half of the baguette and add the cheese, breaking the slices up if you need to.
3. Scatter the pepper, beetroot, radish and carrot along the baguette, then add the leaves, dribble with the pesto and close the baguette.
4. Wrap the baguette tightly in baking parchment and tie securely with string.

5. Take a bread knife with you so you can slice it when you're ready to eat it.

Rainbow rippled meringues

Prepartion time

1 hour 45 minutes

Ingredients

- 4 large eggs whites
- 225g white caster sugar
- Plus three of the following flavours: Lemon meringues
- very finely grated zest 1 lemon

- yellow food colouring paste
- Orange meringues
- very finely grated zest 1 orange
- orange food colouring paste
- Pistachio meringues
- 2 tbsp finely chopped shelled pistachio
- green food colouring paste
- Blueberry meringues
- 2 tbsp freeze-dried blueberry , pounded to a dust using a pestle and mortar
- blue food colouring paste
- Lavender meringues
- ½ tbsp dried lavender , pounded to a dust using a pestle and mortar

- purple food colouring paste
- Raspberry meringues
- 2 tbsp freeze-dried raspberries , pounded to dust using a pestle and mortar
- pink food colouring paste
- You'll also need
- disposable piping bags
- small paintbrush
- extra-large round piping nozzle

Instructions

1. Heat oven to 140C/120C fan/gas 1 and line 2 large baking sheets with baking parchment.

2. First, set up your piping bags. You will need 3 disposable piping bags for the 3 flavours.

3. Using a wet paintbrush, paint lines of undiluted food colouring along the inside of the piping bags.

4. Be quite generous, because you want bold colours.

5. Wash the brush well between each colour so they don't mix.

6. Snip off the end of 1 bag and drop in an extra-large round piping nozzle, then put the bags to one side.

7. Tip the egg whites into a large mixing bowl or table-top mixer – make sure it's grease-free before you start.

8. Whisk the eggs with an electric hand whisk or in your mixer, until they hold soft peaks.

9. Begin adding the sugar 1 tbsp at a time, whisking continuously, until you have a thick and glossy meringue, which will hold up in a stiff peak on the end of the whisk.

10. Divide the meringue into 3 bowls and swirl through your chosen flavourings (to correspond to the piping bag colours). You want to achieve a marbled effect rather than thoroughly mixing it all in.

11. Put the piping bag fitted with your nozzle into a tall glass or jug and roll the piping bag down over the lip of the jug to hold it in place.

12. Fill the bag with the correct flavoured meringue to match the colour in the bag.

13. Lift up and twist the end to seal.

14. Hold the piping bag about 2cm vertically above the baking tray.

15. Apply an even pressure to the bag, slowly lifting the bag as you squeeze, to make a smooth round meringue, approximately 6cm wide.

16. To finish with a nice peak at the top, push down a little on the mixture then quickly pull the nozzle away.

17. Continue until all the mixture in the bag is used up, leaving enough room for the meringues to spread a little.

18. Quickly remove the nozzle, wash it and dry well, then drop in the next piping bag.

19. Continue with the remaining mixtures until it they are all used up and you have 2 trays covered with 3 colours of meringues.

20. Bake for 1 hr, turning the heat down to 120C/100C fan/gas ½ for the final 30 mins.

21. Remove from the oven and cool on wire racks while you make another batch of meringues with the remaining 3 flavours, if you like. Can be made up to a week ahead and kept in an airtight container, or serve with our flavoured creams (see tips, below).

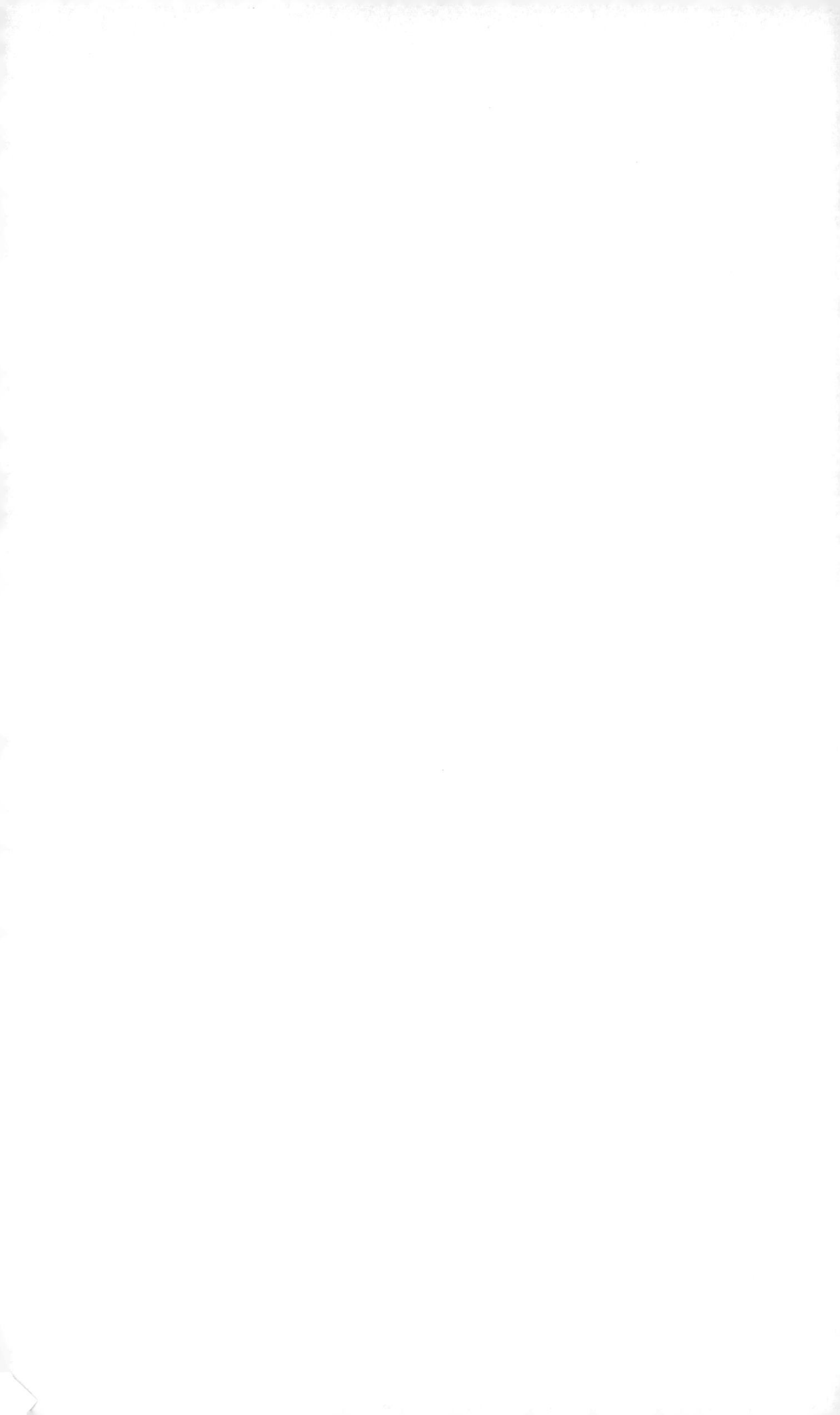

www.ingramcontent.com/pod-product-compliance
Ingram Content Group UK Ltd.
Pitfield, Milton Keynes, MK11 3LW, UK
UKHW022006190726
13853UKWH00004B/1758